ARTIFICIAL HUMAN INSEMINATION

ARTIFICIAL HUMAN INSEMINATION

*

Report of a Conference held in London under the auspices of the Public Morality Council

*

London

WM. HEINEMANN · MEDICAL BOOKS · LTD.

1948

First Published, March, 1947
Reprinted, April, 1948

Printed in Great Britain by
McCorquodale & Co. Ltd., London

FOREWORD

By the Bishop of London

The following record is a factual report of a Conference on Human Artificial Insemination held at the Cowdray Hall, on Thursday, April 11th, 1946. I was not myself present, but I have been asked to write a foreword as President of the Public Morality Council, under whose auspices the Conference was held.

The purpose of the Conference was not to reach conclusions but to uncover as many as possible of the implications of the practice. For this purpose a number of speakers representing different professions and diverse points of view were invited each to state his own side of the case. Law and theology, as well as medicine, were represented; and I think it was surprising to all how many and diverse were the considerations involved.

It should be stated that the Public Morality Council accepts no responsibility for the views expressed by any speaker, nor of course were the speakers themselves responsible for each other's views. The speeches are printed precisely as they were delivered. The organizers of the Conference offer no comment, but hope that from the material thus produced readers may be able to arrive at a balanced judgment of their own.

In conclusion, we should like to offer our thanks, individually and corporately, to Viscount Caldecote for so kindly taking the Chair and to the speakers for the time and trouble they gave to the elucidation of this important and difficult problem.

✠ Wm. Londin.

SECRETARY'S NOTE

It should be understood that the lectures which form this report were prepared for delivery by word of mouth and not with a view to later publication. The conversational form has been retained, but readers will understand that a different style of expression might have been used had our purpose been merely to produce the printed report.

GEORGE TOMLINSON,
General Secretary,
PUBLIC MORALITY COUNCIL.

37, Norfolk Street,
Strand, W.C.2.

CONTENTS

I. THE PROBLEM IN OUTLINE

H. P. NEWSHOLME, M.A., M.D.,
F.R.C.P., B.Sc., D.P.H.

I UNDERSTAND that our purpose to-day is to review procedure and policy in relation to human artificial insemination. My own part is to be that of attempting to provide an outline of the subject sufficient to serve as a framework for use by those who follow me and those who join in the discussion. First, to avoid appearing under false pretences, let me say that on the medical aspect my knowledge is both scanty and wholly second-hand. That is, of course, equally true of the vast majority of the medical profession. The number of those with direct experience in this difficult field must indeed be very restricted. I hope that during the Conference we may have their important contribution and their amplification, or, where necessary, correction of my comments. On other more general aspects, the experience which comes with the passage of the years may, perhaps, allow me to tread more confidently. In a discussion which we all know to be capable of producing warmth beyond the ordinary, I hope to outline the subject as objectively as possible.

First of all, what is human artificial insemination? That preliminary question can conveniently be answered in the clear and short definition which I find in a paper by a group of able exponents of the procedure; . . . " Artificial insemination . . . is the deposition of semen in the vagina, the cervical canal, or the uterus by instruments " . . . and we are now concerned with its utilisation as a method of bringing about pregnancy unattained or unattainable by ordinary sexual union. The procedure for artificial insemination involves a succession of stages and the use of alternative methods. The first step is that of detailed examination of the genital system in both husband and wife, to detect, and, if possible, remove hindrances arising from physical anomalies making for infecundity. There should go with this a general examination aimed at the elimination of psychological difficulties to effective union. This is followed by a fecundity examination in both. The husband's fecundity is reviewed by microscopical inspection of a specimen of semen obtained by masturbation. The examination covers the number, appearance and motility of the sperm cells. So far as the woman is concerned, the degree of penetrability of the wife's genital tract by the sperm cells is examined by the physician, who inseminates her vagina, by means of a syringe, with the sperm procured from the husband by his masturbation. The clear plug of mucus filling the woman's cervix during the ovulatory phase of the menstrual cycle is then sampled, and the sample examined microscopically to ascertain the degree of penetration by the sperm cells. The ovulatory phase is itself previously determined by training the woman to take her rectal temperature in the early morning, the ovulatory phase corresponding with the sudden dip in the temperature to a minimal level. Infecundity may be related to primary scantiness or poor motility or other defect in the sperm cells, or to the chemical or physical obstruction to their progress presented in the woman's genital tract by the cervical mucus plug. I have found no reference to any ascertainment of the fecundity of the ovum itself. This, presumably, is at present incapable of exploration.

Having determined that artificial insemination

shall be applied to aid fertilisation, what various methods can be used? Let us consider, first of all, insemination from husband to wife. There it may be effected according to the circumstances, either by the wife after instruction or by the physician.

In the case of vaginal insemination effected by the wife, the physician teaches the wife the technique of vaginal self-insemination, the semen being produced by the husband by masturbation. The semen is received into a clean dry vessel and then injected by the wife into her own vagina when lying on her back, by means of a syringe, the ovulatory phase of the menstrual cycle being chosen for the operation. I gather that this method can be used where the husband is impotent and thus incapable of penetration, but where he may, nevertheless, be able to provide a fecund semen by masturbation. Conception is said to take place readily

The second method is cervical insemination effected by the physician. This can be carried out in one of two ways. The first method utilises normal sexual union. Within one hour after coitus the wife is seen by the physician who draws up into a syringe a little of the semen left in her vaginal pool from the coitus and injects it further along the cervical canal to enable it to surmount the hurdle of the cervical plug. Under the second method semen is obtained direct from the husband by his masturbation instead of through sexual congress, the physician then injecting the semen by a syringe into the wife's cervical canal. In both methods the insemination is made to coincide with the ovulatory phase. Both methods are reported as being applied to cases of failure by the husband to ejaculate semen effectively or to those of too feeble cervical penetration by the sperm cells.

The second group in artificial insemination is that from donor to wife—what is known as "alien" insemination or A.I.D., the first group being known as A.I.H. or insemination of the wife by her husband. Where the husband is found to be sterile or, apparently on occasion where there is risk of conveyance of some marked hereditary defect, those working in this field have developed a procedure whereby a willing donor of semen is selected as suitable for this purpose, the semen resulting from masturbation collected, and a small amount then inseminated into the woman's cervical canal by the physician's syringe. The donor is selected as being physically healthy, free from transmissible disease of body or mind, or from major genetic weaknesses. He must also be free from notable physical features likely to be recognised in the child. He must be himself fecund, having had at least two children, and must in general terms be well-balanced. He must naturally be willing to donate his sperm, and his wife likewise must be willing for him to do so, and both have to accept that the donation is to be by means of an act of masturbation. Further, the woman to be inseminated and her husband must both not only agree, but actively desire—and they must express that desire in writing—that the services of a donor, by preference personally unknown to them, shall be used. The physician for his part, has to undertake to keep that document, with a parallel one from the donor, safely locked up, with instructions for their destruction unread in the event of his death.

A third group is that of artificial insemination from the donor to spinster or widow. I do not know whether this development of the principle of artificial insemination has passed from theory into practice. If so, it will no doubt follow the same technique as applies to the artificial insemination of the married woman from a donor. Even if it has not yet been practised, correspondence in the medical Press has more than once referred appreciatively to its advantages on the grounds either of meeting the calamity of a dwindling population or of remedying the hardship involved to so many spinsters whom the war has deprived of potential husbands, or to young widows, the victims of that same calamity. The leaflet of advice provided by an agency which deals with the legal protection of medical practitioners in their professional relationships contains a clause which avowedly covers, as a practical possibility, the involvement of the practitioner in the artificial insemination of spinsters or of widows.

From that imperfect outline of the procedure I turn to the question of policy, considering this in relation to the successive methods of insemination which I have enumerated. First of all, artificial insemination from husband to wife. Sterility between a couple devoted to each other and earnestly desiring children is a great calamity. If it is irremediable then the couple must, and can, make the best of it getting fulness of life in other ways. In that respect the familiar phrase in the marriage ceremony as to husband and wife taking each other "for better, for worse" has both a deep comfort and an equally deep significance too easily overlooked by those who expect complete satisfaction as of right, in the absence of which they record the result too hastily as complete failure. Before accepting such a limited scope of marriage, however, the couple are fully justified in seeking every legitimate means of remedy for apparent mutual infecundity. Where husband and wife have fully but fruitlessly explored all the more usual and simple channels of remedy, artificial insemination, suitably applied, is not only legitimate but praiseworthy. It is a troublesome, unromantic and unpleasantly public way of acquiring a family ; but if the couple are prepared to submit themselves to this, their doggedness deserves nothing but admiration.

We have noted three methods of applying artificial insemination from husband to wife—vaginal self-insemination by the wife, cervical insemination effected by the physician from the vaginal pool after normal coitus, and cervical insemination at the physician's hands from the husband's semen produced by masturbation as contrasted with coitus. Can approval be extended to all three methods ? The answer must be related to the circumstance that medical science is being asked to help towards the effective performance of the most fundamental physical function of humanity, the continuance of the human race. That function, however, is as much spiritual as physical, in that it arises out of the blended spiritual and physical relationship of marriage. The help which medical science brings must therefore not involve any element which could lower the dignity of that relationship or of the act of conception which is its climax. I do not hesitate to say that masturbation on the part of the husband, as a necessary antecedent to conception, is emphatically a most signal lowering of that dignity. I have indeed been surprised, in relation to a comment on my part, in the correspondence columns of the medical Press, that this element of masturbation was one specifically to eliminate as " besmirching " to the procedure, to find how positive has been the protest by individual medical men and women against any such assertion, with the counter accusation of prudery and the counter assertion of the lack of significance of the precise manner of production of the semen. Old fashioned though it may be, I continue to believe that the involvement of masturbation in certain stages preliminary to insemination must be an absolute veto on that particular method of application, even where the principle of insemination under the given circumstances may be accepted as legitimate. A fair end may not be attained by foul means ; and the fairness of the end cannot make foul into fair in the means, where these involve a function which all men and all women, past the earliest stage of childhood, universally recognise as the most fundamental one round which their lives as human beings are built.

Therefore I submit that out of the three methods of artificial insemination from husband to wife, two should be rejected—self insemination by the wife and insemination through the physician from semen derived from the husband by masturbation. That leaves, as the only legitimate method at present applicable, so far as is known to me, the insemination of the wife from the vaginal pool after normal coitus.

That takes us back to an earlier stage in the preliminary examination for fecundity, where the husband's semen is obtained by masturbation. The need for that examination arises, I suppose, from a laudable desire on the part of the physician to be as thorough as possible, with, no doubt, the practical purpose also of avoiding the trouble and waste of time of insemination from the husband if, in fact, he is infecund. But is there any reason why, where examination of the wife suggests the course, and where artificial insemination after normal coitus by the couple is then being applied by the physician, this should not be carried out without investigation of the husband's state of fecundity, if such investigation can only be by way of masturbation on his part ? If there is success, well and good. If there is failure after renewed attempts, then the couple have done all possible and the physician has not substantially wasted his time. There should, indeed be no regard given to waste of time if the process by which he would save time implies, as I suggest it does, that the patient is to behave unworthily for the convenience of the physician. That married couples can themselves take such a view is indicated by the naive comment in a paper on the subject, that the theoretical risks of bacterial infection inherent in insemination from the vaginal pool have sometimes to be accepted because "some couples cannot adjust themselves to other methods of obtaining semen." The delicacy of that phrasing seems in itself a notable manifestation of prudery, an unwillingness to draw attention to a spade being a spade; and that very avoidance of downrightness in such a connection seems to me to have a powerful significance.

My own conclusion would be this. First, an absolute refusal to recognise as legitimate any process whether of attainment of fecundity or of effecting artificial insemination which involves masturbation on the part of the husband. Secondly, that in artificial insemination between husband and wife, justified after full exploration of hindrances to conception, only one method so far devised can be countenanced, that of insemination of the wife from the vaginal pool after normal coitus.

The second group is that of alien insemination from donor to wife, from a man other than the husband. On the yardstick which I have already mentioned—quite apart from other considerations—the method stands self-condemned. There is inevitably masturbation by the donor, almost certainly repeated acts of masturbation before conception follows; and masturbation moreover, allowed by the donor's wife as being a necessary party to the donation. There are other obvious considerations weighing against the legitimacy of alien insemination. The donor, as we have seen, is chosen as appearing to be healthy and otherwise suitable. It seems to me to be a remarkable act of faith on the part of the physician to regard any particular donor with confidence as a reliable and desirable sire for the child whom the couple wish to have. It would appear that the same donor is, on occasion, utilised for a succession of alien inseminations, and he may be one of a panel of donors used systematically to provide a semen "bank." I find myself looking with distaste on the curious qualities of the man willing to serve in such a capacity, and still more at the very willingness to act as father at a distance to a progeny he will not know, by a process which involves him in repeated schoolboy tricks, with the added indignity of the wife's compliance. I hope that this peculiar temperament would not be one to be bequeathed to the proposed posterity, for it seems neither a desirable nor a normal masculine trait.

Then there are disquieting legal aspects. The physician is not exempt from the rules of morality applying to men at large, and to these the bearing of a child by a woman to a man not her husband constitutes in principle a deed of adultery, even though the physical act of adultery has been avoided. I do not pretend to know the verdict at which the law might arrive; but the law would certainly have something to say on this pseudo-adultery, and the legal liabilities are viewed with disquiet by those who have considered the position. That is clearly reflected in the leaflet of advice issued by a medical protection society to those of its members who seek information on the subject. There are other considerable complications in regard to the legitimacy of the child, and of his inheritance of the husband's property on the latter's decease, even though not actually the child of that man, not to mention those other quite possible complications following on a transiently complacent husband repenting too late of his consent and treating the child as a bastard.

Even if the law should rule that the child is not illegitimate in the absence of proof of non-access, there is still the awkwardness, from the legal standpoint, of a birth certificate which either omits the husband's name from the description of the child's parentage or else falsely enters him as the father. The law will undoubtedly have much to say. Whatever its decisions, my own clear conviction is that alien artificial insemination, that is insemination from a donor, cannot be justified under any circumstances. It is a perversion of the meaning of marriage, capable of being adopted only where the Christian idea of marriage as a life-long, completely exclusive consecration to each other of one man and one woman, to the absolute bar of all others, has been rejected in its essential principle.

I turn finally and briefly to the third group, the insemination of the unmarried or of the widow. That sounds an improbable and, indeed, a preposterous development, but as I have already mentioned, correspondence in the medical Press has shown quite an appreciable sprinkling of opinion favouring the artificial insemination, on request, of spinsters or widows. I gather, in correspondence with the secretary of a medical advisory organisation, that his governing Committee have received an inquiry on the matter, and have not regarded compliance by the practitioner with a request for such insemination as of itself constituting dishonourable professional action. That seems to be a remarkable conclusion. I do not see how, to those who are prepared to tolerate such procedure, marriage can have any real significance at all, or man seem more than a superior type of animal. The recognition of the spiritual element in marriage, the element of discipline as contrasted with the element of emotionalism which appears to overwhelm the advocates of alien insemination, is essential if the humanitarianism which leads to the invention of these ingenious devices is not to play havoc where it is intended to bring a blessing. Whatever the reports—and they are, of course, forthcoming—of the happiness in marriage to which a child born by alien insemination is found to give rise, I am convinced that cumulative experience, if, unhappily, it is allowed to accumulate, will show eventually how fundamentally the procedure weakens the marriage bond.

Questions and Answers

1. Does Dr. Newsholme consider the practice of testing the fecundity of the man by examination of a specimen from the vaginal pool after normal coitus to be morally objectionable ?

A. I see no objection to that at all because it arises from the ordinary processes of marriage.

Q. Can it be explained how there can be any medical treatment of sterility if the criterion is taken that any examination of the life of the male sperm is beneath the dignity of the couple ? Why should the women have to be operated on and bear all the brunt of the investigation when it is known that in nine cases out of ten it is the male who is infecund ? Is it suggested that there should be no serious treatment of barren women?

A. That is not my feeling at all. I see no reason why the doctor should not go to a great deal of trouble in helping both husband and wife to become fecund; but that must be subject to the dignity of their relations to one another. I said that to many couples this way of settling their problem is so undignified that they are not prepared to undergo it. I think the medical profession has got to accept a limitation on its great powers, a limitation from the ideals of marriage itself.

Q. I spend a great deal of my time in trying to ascertain the fertility of a husband in order that when he is responsible for the absence of a family the wife shall not be subjected, perhaps, to major operations, or at any rate to a great deal of unnecessary treatment. Is my work to be regarded as entirely superfluous?

A. Surely you will not expect me to reply to that.

Q. Dr. Newsholme does not consider it morally objectionable to take a specimen of semen after normal coitus in order to inject it into the cervical canal, yet he considers that there is an objection to examination of semen under a microscope. Is there not some inconsistency?

A. These are not identical operations at all. For the husband to deposit semen in the wife's vagina is normal procedure. Masturbation, on the other hand, is not normal procedure.

II. MEDICAL

By Kenneth Walker, F.R.C.S.

I am not going to speak for the medical profession; no speaker can represent the views of the medical profession. I speak as an individual. Perhaps the chief difference between Dr. Newsholme and myself is that I have spent a great many years of my life in the study of human fertility whilst he speaks only from a perusal of its medical literature. I have, of course, no practical experience of artificial insemination, because that is the work of the Gynæcologist, but much experience of the men and women who ask that insemination should be carried out. Let me assure you that medical men and women are not light-hearted in their adoption of this method. Instinctively one revolts from such an artificial method of continuing the human race, for it is far too reminiscent of that materialistic, ultra-scientific "brave new world" that Aldous Huxley once painted for us, to be pleasing. We would avoid it whenever possible yet many of us feel that in certain circumstances, and under certain conditions, it is justifiable. There is no unanimity in the medical profession on this subject; you have already observed that today. I personally disagree profoundly with the previous speaker.

I am not going to talk about artificial insemination with the husband's semen. I will assume that where the husband is incurably impotent, the majority of people will agree that the wife should not be deprived of the possibility of having a child because the husband, although fertile, is impotent. I am going to talk about the vexed question of artificial insemination by donated semen. I know nothing at all about the artificial insemination of spinsters and widows; that is a subject which is entirely new to me, so I shall limit myself to the subject of donated semen when the husband is incurably sterile. As Dr. Newsholme has rightly said, we would only consider carrying out insemination when both parties had considered the matter very carefully and had agreed that they wanted it to be done. It occasionally happens that either the husband or the wife comes to the doctor and says that he or she would like it to be carried out without the knowledge of the other. They do not ask this for unworthy motives; the wife may wish to spare her husband humiliation, and the husband may have an equally good reason for making the request. But on no account will any doctor have anything to do with such an arrangement. Unless both parties agree to insemination it is never carried out.

There are various ways in which the opponents of artificial insemination of donated semen argue against it. One is the well known method *reductio ad absurdum.* A picture is drawn of insemination being carried out on such a wide scale that it becomes a general substitute for normal intercourse. It was even suggested at a recent meeting, at which I was not present, that unscrupulous doctors might inseminate women with Chinese semen! I have a very high appreciation of China, but if arguments are to carried out on those lines, where are we going to get? Let us try to be more practical and reasonable than this. It is quite possible that doctors might sometimes abuse their power, for insemination is putting a great deal of power in their hands. But you have got to remember that you trust the surgeon who operates on you and it would be very easy for him to kill you instead of trying to cure you. If you trust us with you lives I think it is reasonable to suppose that we will not play all those criminal tricks which some of the opponents of insemination fear. I agree that it is putting a great deal of power into our hands. Look at the possibilities, for example, in a case in which the inheritance of a large estate or of a title is concerned. There is no heir, the husband is subfertile, and it is suggested that insemination should be carried out with his semen in the hope of increasing his wife's chances of bearing a child. What is to prevent the inseminator from using, not the husband's semen, but some highly fertile semen from another source? It is perhaps unfortunate that you have to put such confidence in the medical profession and it is possible that on rare occasions insemination will be abused. That is a risk which has to be accepted.

Let me make my position clear. I am not a gynæcologist and never in my life have I carried out insemination. I am supposed to be an expert in male fertility and if Dr. Newsholme is to be believed, I have wasted 20 years of my life. It is my responsibility to see the husband and to say whether a husband is infertile. After seeing the husbands I generally see the wives. I should like now to talk about some of the psychological objections which are brought forward against insemination. A man has every right to say that the practice is unethical, immoral and un-Christian, but unfortunately opponents of insemination weaken their case by producing armchair psychological arguments against it. It is said, for instance, that the method weakens the marriage bond and that the husband might just as well encourage his wife to take a lover. But the position is quite different. The intervention of a lover, a human figure who the wife knows to be the father of her child, completely alters the situation. This might very well weaken the wife's feeling for her husband but it is not likely that a purely scientific procedure like insemination will have the same effect. Actually, I have seen many marriages saved by the arrival of a child, an event for which the wife has been longing for years. Another thing which has impressed me has been the rapidity with which the husband forgets that the child is not his. Within a comparatively short time he begins to talk about it as though it were his own child. I have seen many more marriages saved rather than wrecked by the procedure of artificial insemination. It may be said that the same end might be achieved by adoption. I do not know if you have had any experience of finding a child for a childless couple to adopt. There is a tremendous demand for children ; they will not go round. It must also be remembered that there is the fundamental association in a woman's mind between her child and labour, a thing which is never quite satisfied by the adoption of a child, although adoption is extremely successful in the majority of cases.

I have always noticed when I have talked on this subject that it is the men who are the chief objectors, and I am inclined to think that this is because a man does not really realise the longing of a childless woman for a child. It is very easy to say that a couple have married and have taken each other for better or worse and that if the husband turns out to be sterile they will have to accept this fact. But when a woman longs for a child and hopes for it for years and years and it never comes, the longing may reach such intensity as to spoil the whole of her life. Dr. Newsholme said that he spoke not as one with direct knowledge of this subject, but, as I understood him, more from the theoretical point of view. He regards insemination in any form and on any occasion as immoral and for him the whole subject turns on the question of masturbation.

I do not want to deal with such an unsavoury subject. I can only say that I, who have to deal with the sexual difficulties of the male, find that much of my work is the direct result of the tremendous stress which is laid on the deadly sin of masturbation. It has been the custom—and I am afraid that teachers and the clergy are often, in my opinion, guilty of this—to try to cure boys of masturbation by telling them of the dreadful things that will happen to them in future years as a result of it. The number of neurotics and impotent husbands I see later, who are frightened that they have ruined themselves for life as a result of masturbation, is tremendous. I have even seen young men rendered suicidal as the result of this stupid and pernicious teaching and I am sure that some otherwise inexplicable suicides have been amongst its fruits.

I do not want to trespass on the theologians' province, but let me say that we recognise that the religious aspect is extremely important. We live in an age in which expediency takes precedence over morality. For a great good a little evil is very readily done and the strong teaching of Christ is watered down to suit our palates. I only say this in order to emphasise the fact that I appreciate the religious aspect of this subject. I attended a meeting at Oxford at which Dr. Russell was Chairman and to my surprise the theologians were much more restrained in their comments on insemination than many of the doctors I have encountered. Never have I heard the subject discussed with so little passion. The views put forward were naturally based on the teaching of the Church from the time of St. Paul to Thomas Aquinas, namely, that marriage was for the purpose of satisfaction of the sexual needs of the marriage partners and for the propagation of children. The view was expressed that these two activities must never be separated and that insemination therefore could not be tolerated. It was immoral to separate the reproductive function from the sexual function. I should like to point out that if that is an objection then the Anglican Church cannot countenance the use of birth control, where the reproductive function is isolated from the sexual function. The Oxford theologians were—some of them—inclined to support artificial insemination by means of the husband's semen when the husband is impotent and cannot perform the sexual act. Again, in that case there is a separation of the two functions.

Artificial insemination is a discovery in science and we all know from the example of the discovery of atomic energy that scientific discoveries may be used for evil as well as for good. I have agreed that this discovery may be easily abused. I agree that it has got to be safeguarded, but I am of the opinion that it is often justifiable because it will bring into many homes happiness where unhappiness previously existed, and tend not to destroy but to safeguard the marriage.

Questions and Answers

Q. Can you tell me if Hippocrates had anything to say on the subject of masturbation ? He is regarded as the moral leader of the medical profession.

A. I am afraid that I know nothing of Hippocrates's view on the subject. He wrote on so many important subjects that this must have escaped his attention.

Q. Since the procedure with regard to artificial insemination depends almost entirely on the incapacity of the infecund husband, can Mr. Walker say what proportion of husbands are in that category ? and what possibilities he envisages may be available in the development of medical science in the future to remedy that infecundity ?

A. It is impossible to obtain figures. As I have spent my time in seeing a selected group of husbands I may have an exaggerated view of the prevalence of infertility in males. It has been said that in about one-third of the cases of voluntary childless marriages the husband is mainly at fault and in two-thirds of the cases he is a factor in the childlessness. It is often the case that children do not arrive, not because the husband or wife is completely sterile, but because there are sterility factors on both sides. The difficulty of separating out these cases and of producing figures will therefore be appreciated.

Infertility is extremely common in this country and the cause is often unknown. It may be that there are factors in our modern civilisation which render the man less fertile. The treatment of the infertile male is also, as yet, very imperfect.

Q. Anyone with experience of dealing with youths and young men knows that very frequently harm has been done by exaggerating to them the future results of masturbation. Does Mr. Walker feel that there is a fundamental moral objection to masturbation, even for purposes of artificial insemination ?

A. I must answer No. If it is done deliberately, without feelings of guilt, for the purpose of a wife obtaining a child, I cannot see any moral objection.

Q. From a purely scientific point of view, if the practice of insemination became very common, and applied chiefly to people of lesser fecundity, would it not be harmful eugenically from the point of view of the community as a whole ?

A. An argument can be put forward in favour of that point on theoretical grounds but there is no reason to believe that infecundity is inherited. I used to make enquiries of the infertile male about his family but I found there was no relationship between the fertility of the parents and that of the children and I have given up taking family history into account.

III. SOCIOLOGICAL

By Professor E. O. James

With regard to the sociological approach to the problem, it should be examined in its cultural context in relation to three things :—

(1) The parents who are involved in the practice.
(2) Family life.
(3) Society as a whole.

Biologically speaking, the continuity of the race could be secured perfectly well by the casual mating of the male and female as and when required and desired for the purpose of producing offspring. But there is a great deal more in the human relationship of husband and wife than the mere mating of male and female for the production of offspring. Human society, whatever the Marxists and others may have said, never has been promiscuous. Of that I feel perfectly certain, speaking as an anthropologist. The human infant requires prolonged care. This produces a parental impulse and as a result the male and the female human species are conscious of being related to one another in a peculiarly intimate relationship, for the purpose of reproducing the race in an orderly manner and for the mutual care of each other and of the offspring. All this presupposes a family relationship based upon a sound marriage system in which the union between man and wife is deepened and expressed in sexual intercourse.

The aim of sexual intercourse is twofold. In the first place it is to consolidate the nuptial union and therefore to promote harmony in the home. Secondly, it is to procreate children and so ensure the continuance of the family and the permanence of the family unit. Anything which upsets this very carefully balanced equilibrium is anti-social and it is because of this that marriage has been surrounded with very carefully prescribed rules and prohibitions in order to prevent disorderly relationships, sexual jealousies and anything which might disturb the peace and harmony of the home. These sanctions which, of course, are not peculiar to Christianity or our own system, being a universal phenomena throughout the whole of the human social organisation, are not just meaningless taboos. They have grown up for a particular sociological purpose, namely, the protection of the home and of family life at its most vital point. Once the family as the nucleus of human society breaks up, the whole social structure disintegrates. There are abundant evidences of this, not least at the present time.

Sociologically, the problem is to consider how far, if at all, the practice of artificial insemination conflicts with any of the safeguards to the cohesion and solidarity of the family and of the home. Speaking from this point of view—and I am not concerned with the ethical, or with the theological aspects of the practice at the moment—what we commonly call A.I.H. (artificial insemination from the husband) does not raise a serious issue, though, as previous speakers have shown, the situation is very different in the moral and religious sphere.

Passing to A.I.D. the sociological implications are by no means negligible. The husband is placed in very much the same position that he occupied in a matriarchal state of society when there was a widespread ignorance of the physiological facts in regard to paternity and when the husband was regarded merely as the man who was married to a woman who produced children. But she gave birth to children not through and by him since it was supposed that the function of the father was merely to open the way for some spirit-child to enter the woman and so for an ancestor to be re-incarnated. The husband was not, therefore, regarded as the actual father of the child. He was merely there in the capacity of a guardian or protector, both of the woman and of the offspring. His function was to facilitate the entrance of the "spirit-child" into the woman. The infant was regarded purely as the production of the mother, so that between the father and the child there was no vital point of union. Indeed, the father had no social definition at all. All the contacts were with the mother and with her relations. The child was often brought up under the authority of her brother, his uncle, and the father took no real and active part in its education and training.

I quote this example from a more primitive state of culture because it has some bearing upon our present problem inasmuch as it shows, in the absence of adequate sociological data concerning the practice of Artificial Insemination in modern civilized communities, the effect upon the family and society (admittedly organised on a very different basis) of the elimination of the paternal functions of the lawful father in nuptial relationships. Under matriarchal conditions, when the husband ceased to be regarded as the real and actual progenitor of his offspring, paternal authority and responsibility were seriously undermined, and, notwithstanding the many safeguards that were introduced to keep the family unit intact, the practice unquestionably had a disintegrating influence upon the whole social structure. It seems, in fact, to have been an important contributory cause of the break-up of this type of society. So in the case of A.I.D. where a not wholly dissimilar set of circumstances might well prevail if the custom became normal. Here again the husband-wife relation is fundamentally disorganised by the introduction of a third party in the form of the donor, so that the lawful spouse, not theoretically but *actually*, has no part or lot in the procreation of the child or children who are born by this method to his wife.

The sociological complications of such a situation are obvious. Apart from the fact that incestuous unions might be contracted in this way if and when the donor were a near relative, the disruptive effect upon family solidarity is inevitable. The offspring would be no longer the fruit of the procreative relationship between husband and wife as co-partners in the establishment of their family. The children would be deprived of a natural father whose paternal care, affection and authority could hardly fail to be jeopardised by a wholly fictitious and unnatural state of affairs, harmful alike to all concerned—husband, wife, children and the community at large. Moreover, the sexual act would lose its romantic significance and be reduced to a mechanical process in which marriage need play no part at all, and if the practice were extended to spinsters and widows—indeed, to all and sundry—as has been foreshadowed, a state of promiscuity would result.

Therefore, in its sociological and cultural implications, A.I.D. appears to stand condemned equally in respect of its effects on (1) conjugal solidarity and paternal control (2) the cohesion of family life and harmony in the home (3) since the family is the nucleus of society, on the social structure as an integrated whole dependent upon a healthy and harmonious family organisation.

Questions and Answers

Q. Has Professor James any information respecting the American figures? I believe that there are 5,000 tabulated cases and the results have shown an alteration in the balance of the sexes. A.I.D. seems to produce a ratio of 150 males to 100 females.

A. It is difficult to get at this kind of information, but should it affect the proportion of male and female, sociologically this would be a matter of the most vital importance.

IV. PSYCHOLOGICAL

By William Brown, D.M.(Oxon.), D.Sc. (Lond.), F.R.C.P.

As a medical psychologist, I cannot say much about A.I.D. but I can say something about A.I.H. because at least one of my patients has received treatment in that way. Her husband had lost potency to a partial extent and as a young wife with an older husband she was very anxious to have a child. She went through what was to her the unpleasant process of artificial insemination from her husband. So I have been able to form an empirical psychological opinion in at least one case. Psychologically, we know that the family has been the fundamental unit since very remote times and that that situation has left its mark on the mind of man, so that the little child comes into the world with arche-type reactions which are related to the history of the race, quite apart from inherited characteristics. Any alteration in the production of children will be bound to have repercussions, but one cannot say that it will necessarily be bad. It will be disturbing at first. When speakers point to the disturbing effect sociologically, it should be remembered that one very great philosopher, perhaps the greatest of ancient times, advocated community of wives and children. Plato, in his " Republic" took a great deal of trouble in working that method out and I should like to see many more people read that book. It should be extensively read, as well as the Gospels, in this age of transition.

But as a medical psychologist of thirty years practice, who has had the opportunity to observe the mind directly in the consulting room—the most important source of knowledge of patients being that obtained during a long series of sittings—I feel quite certain in my own mind that anything of this sort will have serious psychological repercussions. I think that as a medical psychologist and physician, only under very special conditions would one countenance it at all, quite apart from the ethical and religious points of view. From the strictly psychological point of view I would, at any rate, limit it within the family. If the woman is married I would limit artificial insemination to a special situation in which the father is impotent or where there are other reasons why he is unable to be the father of any children born to that woman. It must be remembered that even the mere knowledge of the existence of the donor will have a strong effect on the prospective mother and therefore upon the state of mind she is in while bearing the child.

Inheritance of acquired characteristics has not been proved, although a great deal of work has been carried out on the subject. Professor Wm. McDougall was quite certain that he had proved the existence of acquired characteristics by experiments on rats. However that may be, we are completely in the dark as yet upon the emotional effect—the effect that the emotions in the expectant mother will have on the growing child. Physiologically and anatomically we know that the two are separate before birth except that there is an osmotic interchange in the separated blood streams of mother and child as the child develops its various vital systems, the nervous system being particularly important. The workings of the sympathetic nervous system, in theory at least, produce changes which will modify the development of the child. If the mother is in a normal condition and is hopefully looking forward to having a child she is prepared to love, it may have a beneficial effect on the child. Many people, however, say that it will have no effect whatever. The fact is that we do not know. As a responsible doctor and scientist I say that we simply do not know and so we cannot act as if we did know, but we should keep our minds open to the *possibility* of the emotional effect of this practice on the mother in relation to the child.

But apart from that, and besides the reaction of the father of the family to this knowledge, which he should and must have—I mean if there is a husband in the case—there is a special psychological situation involved. There are at least two people involved, and when the child comes there is a third. When the child comes, it comes with the father-image in its mind. There is no doubt that the child will speculate about who its father is. Little children do that although the parents do not know about it. We know that from the analytic experience we have of our patients. It is extraordinary how intelligent a child can be until its intelligence is inhibited by repression. The little child is intelligent and its intelligence goes in a particular direction. It is always speculating where it came from and how it was born. No doubt, in relation to artificial insemination, it will be told that the husband is its father but in time the truth will leak out. I have seen that happen with adopted children. The question arises; when should the boy or girl be told he or she is an adopted child? When the child is told it is a severe mental shock, sometimes being quite disastrous.

I am quite sure that artificial insemination is not needed except in very special cases, and those special cases can look after themselves until later on when we know more than we do at present about insemination. It may be asked how can we know what will happen until we have tried. There is nothing so stupid in the world but that some people are ready and eager to try it. Although I listened with great interest to Professor

James's sociological difficulties I could not help feeling that a good many of the sociological rules and customs he mentioned have been based on ignorance and sheer guess-work. We must build up our ideas in relation to modern scientific knowledge and we should not be too ready to brush aside a new venture. That is another matter. But one is right in considering the controversy, so long as it is a controversy based on the actual working of the mind, as still unsettled.

Questions and Answers

Q. Does Dr. Brown consider that if artificial insemination became widespread and almost on a par with ordinary creative working, there is, say, possibility of new vices and crime arising?

A. I think that is quite possible. Personally I doubt if this process will be adopted to any extent. I think it is more likely to be a temporary process, because the strong feelings in relation to sex and normal heterosexuality are the means of keeping society level and on an even keel. If the process did become extensively used, we should begin to have the conditions of Plato's "Republic" coming into being—a movement towards community of wives and children. One might have to alter the structure of society, but to my mind that is not likely to happen until the Christian religion is stamped out and the majority of people say that there is nothing in religion and that science is the only God—which is absurd.

Q. The speaker suggests that a woman who is artificially inseminated will feel disturbed during pregnancy. What would be the feelings of the same woman if she has to go childless when the greatest object of her marriage is the idea of bearing children? What bearing would that have upon the union of two people ?

A. That is a fundamental question. There are other ways in which a woman who is childless can acquire children. Divorce is supposed to be justified in the circumstances outlined. Nullity of marriage is allowed by the Roman Catholic Church in such cases.

Q. The speaker suggests that the practice of artificial insemination is not likely to be widespread in the future. Can that statement be supported when we are living in a sociological *milieu* which is driving people towards artificial insemination through building up in the minds of married people a strong conception of the value of the family ? Means are being provided by which young couples can determine quite easily whether they are likely to have a family. Are we not driving people to feel that marriage is not complete unless they have children ?

A. No doubt these are possibilities. Medical examination before marriage might help and it must be remembered that nullity decrees and divorce are possible. Where there is a sterile marriage, there is a strong natural pull away from the situation after a time, however friendly the couple may still be.

V. THEOLOGICAL
(The Roman Catholic Church)

By The Rev. J. C. Heenan, D.D.

Whenever scientific problems arise requiring an expression of theological opinion there is a danger lest truth be obscured through prejudice. By prejudice I mean, oddly enough, not the prejudice of conservative Christians, but rather the prejudice of those who know well that Galileo was condemned by the Church and that certain bishops frowned on anæsthetics, but are quite unaware that the overwhelming majority of the pioneers of science were believing and practising Christians. I think it is necessary to say that by way of preamble because I have no intention whatever of apologising for the very strict and, indeed, rigid views which the Catholic Church holds and teaches on moral questions. It is not too much to say that the one fear which seems to infect the otherwise intrepid Church of Rome is a fear of being thought broad-minded. The Church recoils quite instinctively from the ideas of those who describe themselves (and are even described by others) as progressives. When I say that the Church recoils, I am referring to the perfectly spontaneous reaction of Catholics in every part of the world and of all conditions. We know that there is such a thing as mass enthusiasm and mass decision. In Moscow, workers recoil to order from Fascist beasts, whether they are disguised as earnest Christians or Ernest Bevins. What we need to know is whether the instinctive reactions of Catholics against many modern ethical developments are based on sound principles or are merely thoughtless judgments of the minds of a laity atrophied because all thinking on moral questions is conducted exclusively on their behalf by a celibate clergy.

A ready example is to be found in contraception. Forward thinking, progressive men, hold that in certain circumstances artificial birth prevention is a counsel of wisdom. Catholics hold that it is " masturbation *a deux* " and, as such, intrinsically wrong. No Catholic denies that the coming of children may be highly inconvenient to the purse of the father or to the health of the mother. Mr. Walker has referred to masturbation and has said that he has met many whose lives have been ruined through the dreadful things said by teachers of the horrible results of masturbation. The facts in relation to priests are that an earlier generation of doctors did hold that masturbation caused these unhappy results and the priests, being always docile to the medical profession, taught what they had been told to teach.

Many Catholics no doubt practise birth prevention. Many more would like to do so. The same is true, perhaps, of adultery. Sin is almost always attractive ; that is why it is dangerous. A man who practises self-denial at certain times when living with his wife or, as a soldier on active service, denies himself for years, may be laughed at by his friends and sneered at by intellectuals but he will be commended by the Church, and, as we believe, by Christ Himself.

I hope that you do not despair of my coming to the point of this discussion. I assure you that it is highly necessary for me to accentuate the unattractive, if characteristic, outlook of the Catholic on many medico-moral problems. The Church is prepared to be labelled reactionary but she never wants to regret having given enthusiastic support to new schemes for social amelioration. This Conference has been called by the Public Morality Council. A special Sub-Committee is unanimously of the opinion that artificial insemination of the wife by her husband is an entirely personal matter and that religious, moral, social and legal issues are not involved. It will, perhaps, be some preparation for the Catholic Church's strong rebuttal of the artificial insemination under consideration—that is, by donor—if I say that the opinion of the Sub-Committee in question might not have been so unanimous had there been a Catholic taking part in the discussions.

From the Catholic point of view there can be no doubt whatever of the morality of assisted insemination of the wife after normal intercourse with her husband. That is common theological teaching. It is not only permissible but extremely desirable that marital intercourse, for some reason unfruitful, should be perfected by medical skill. This may take the form of preparing the vagina beforehand in order to overcome the obstacle caused by the malformation of the organ and so make it possible for the seed to pass. Alternatively, it may take the form of medical intervention after normal intercourse to assist the deposited seed towards its natural objective. This is common and certain Catholic teaching. To what extent other methods of insemination of wife by husband are morally permissible is disputed among theologians. It is perhaps wise to give at once the Catholic view on matrimonial consent. This is defined in Canon 1081, Section 2, as " an act of the will by which each partner gives and receives permanent and exclusive bodily rights (*ius in corpus*) for the performance of acts fitted of their very nature (*per se*) for the generation of children." Vermeersch, perhaps the greatest moral theologian of our time, held that any artificial insemination of wife by husband is lawful provided that the semen be not wrongly obtained. The manner in which the semen is obtained is a matter of great moment to Catholic theologians. I think it is impossible for anybody to appreciate the Catholic viewpoint on this subject who does not understand the horror in which the Catholic is taught to hold mortal sin.

Mortal sin is something just as real as virtue. According to Catholic teaching there is no advantage in the world which would justify the commission of one grievous sin. A husband is, therefore, not allowed to practise masturbation in order to provide semen. The contrary opinion is recorded in Ballerini Opus Morale, Volume I, No. 1304, and Bernardi Praxis Confessarii, Volume I, No. 1009, which admits the lawfulness of solitary pollution for the purpose of insemination, since there is no frustration of nature, but that view is not held to-day by any recognised author.

It may be admitted that because of the great authority of Vermeersch it is permissible for Catholics to hold, with him, the lawfulness of artificial insemination properly so-called, under certain conditions, but the majority of authors of moral textbooks deny the lawfulness of artificial insemination as such, allowing only what we have described as assisted insemination. The reason why this view is taken by the majority is given by Cappello in "De Sacramentis" Volume 3, Part I, No. 383: "Artificial fecundation properly so called is unlawful in whatever way it is practised for the reason that the natural act of marriage is the copula or the coming together of husband and wife with the object of the procreation of children to be obtained *naturali modo*." Marital concourse, in other words, is a vital act. Assisted insemination is held by all theologians to be allowable because the natural copula takes place.

A minor, though by no means unimportant, point to

consider is this: Marriage is consummated and the impediment of impotence removed by the use of assisted insemination. This is not true of artificial insemination properly so called. This is an added reason why Catholic Canonists are cautious about accepting the lawfulness of artificial insemination of wife by husband irrespective of the method by which the result be achieved.

We now come, rather reluctantly, to the point at issue, namely, the morality of artificial insemination by donor. I say "reluctantly" because from the Catholic side there is so little to be said. The practice is condemned unanimously and unconditionally by Catholic theologians. For this reason there is little to be found in our textbooks beyond the statement of the unlawfulness of this form of insemination. The official reply of the Holy Office to the question: "Is the artificial fecundation of women permissible?" was a laconic "Non licere." It is fairly certain that the Holy Office was considering only the impregnation of a wife by her husband. It is also probable that the reason for the condemnation was the presumed impossibility of obtaining semen save by sinful means. It is most unlikely that theologians of the last century—and this reply of the Holy Office was published on March 24th, 1897—foresaw the present proposal of insemination by donor or, indeed, any of the scientific splendours which we of the atomic age are destined to enjoy. Beyond noting that it is not lawful, Catholic theologians say little about artificial insemination by donor. It is an example of the instinctive reaction to which I made earlier reference. Typical of the Catholic view is the following extract from a speech made by Cardinal Griffin to the Catholic doctors of his diocese in 1944: "After the successful experiments on artificial insemination of cattle, there are voluntary clinics which are attempting the same experiments on human beings. The very mention of such a practice is revolting, but we must be quite clear what we mean by human artificial insemination. I do not refer to what I should describe as assisted insemination of the wife after normal intercourse with her husband. We are concerned with the practice of the artificial insemination of a wife with the seed of a man who is not her husband. Such practice offends against the dignity of man, sins against the law of nature and is unjust to the offspring. The donor of the seed is reduced to the status of a stallion. Further, the usual method by which the seed is obtained, namely, by pollution, is gravely sinful even if obtained from the husband. The act of the wife in receiving the seed of one who is not her husband has the malice of adultery. Let us face facts. This practice is against the natural moral law, by which the procreation of a child takes place within a family and the father of the child undertakes the duties of the upbringing of his progeny. No consent of husband and wife can remove the immorality from the act. I trust that the medical profession will oppose the production of what have been described as test-tube babies, and the attempt to stud-breed human beings. The practice of human artificial insemination was condemned by the Church in 1897 and a Catholic doctor will therefore not be a party to such an operation. This is but a brief statement of the Catholic teaching."

Not to pose a question is not, of course, to be ignorant of how the question should be posed. It is not difficult to see why, according to Catholic principles, it was never thought necessary to raise the issue of Christian wives seeking pregnancy except through their husbands. If parents have not been blessed with children, to use the old-fashioned phrase, and if through the lawful method of fecundation I have described they are unable to have children, the obvious course is to adopt them. Against that is the desire of a woman, herself to bear children. We take it for granted that *pari passu* with the artificial insemination of the woman there be considered the case of a husband of a sterile wife. He might have an equal desire for inseminating some other woman of his choice. If a woman has the natural longing to be a mother the man, presumably, has a natural longing to be a father. In principle, I take it, there is nothing to choose between the two. The Catholic theological viewpoint is so simple and straightforward as to sound almost naïve. It is that the contract of marriage is the giving and accepting of the *ius in corpus* and because it is exclusive it is unthinkable that either wife or husband shall give or receive the fruits of intercourse with any other person.

It is important to stress that beyond the condemnation by the Holy Office, the possibility of a Christian acceptance of the artificial insemination by a donor has not been thought sufficiently controversial to merit much discussion in Catholic circles. As every philosopher knows, the consensus of informed opinion, if not a criterion of truth, is at least a remarkable testimony of a sound tradition. When a reaction is, if I may use the phrase, so universal, it must obviously correspond to a fundamental conviction of the Catholic mind. It is permissible for us to enquire as to the nature of that conviction. It is, first of all, that this new system is degrading to womanhood. It might be merely because hitherto we have been used to talking only of the insemination of animals that we tend to think of insemination as reducing women to the status of cattle. If that were so, it would be merely an emotional reaction. But it is much more than that. It is not likely that true family unity can best be achieved where only the woman is the parent of the children. The wife's test-tube children would be the husband's artificial step-children. I find it hard to believe that mutual love of the partners in marriage would be increased more by artificial insemination of the wife than by adoption whereby husband and wife equally share the joy of legal parenthood.

The joy of the potential father over his inseminated spouse is too reminiscent of Bertrand Russell to command uncritical conviction. I remember where Russell, in " Marriage and Morals," talks about the Trobriand islanders. Quoting Malinowski, he tells us that when an islander has been away on a voyage for a year or more and finds on his return that his wife has a new-born child, he is delighted and quite unable to understand the hints of Europeans suggesting doubts as to his wife's virtue. We cannot, of course, all lay claim to the simple, unaffected faith of a Bertrand Russell. That is, perhaps, why many cannot imagine artificial insemination having the desirable effect of bringing husband and wife closer together.

Catholic theologians have not disputed over this question because to them all this insemination is only adultery at one remove. It does not seem tenable, from the purely philosophical point of view, that a woman is not wrong in accepting pregnancy from a stranger simply because she derives no pleasure from the act whereby she is impregnated. It might almost seem as though the protagonists of insemination were killjoys in preventing normal insemination. It might be argued —and I assure you that I am not being facetious—that a tolerant husband should give permission for his wife to have natural intercourse with the man who is destined to become the father of his (the husband's) legal child. A man has the right to know exactly what type of man is chosen for the father of his wife's child. We need not know a great deal about heredity to appreciate the enormous influence the character of the father would play in the mental and spiritual composition of the artificial baby.

Whatever steps it is proposed to take in order that husband and wife should know all about the character of the donor, it seems to me singularly dangerous in so intimate a matter if their knowledge is only second-hand. But how a more personal acquaintance is possible without the further danger of more formal adultery it is difficult to see. In proportion as a person is worthy to be what is, after all, a human stallion, he would need to be a fine physical specimen. It seems the more desirable, therefore, that prospective parents should personally assure themselves that his moral character is no less perfect.

I leave to others the more obvious difficulties created by the legal consequences of artificial insemination. Canon law has made no pronouncement for the simple reason that theologians have not created the raw material upon which pronouncements may be made. It is clear, however, that to safeguard the institution of marriage, elaborate precautions would have to be taken to remove the danger of consanguinity. This, and other legal points, will no doubt be mentioned later. It remains for me to say, in conclusion, how much I regret having to read a paper which must sound so very reactionary. I do not, of course, regret the attitude of the Church. I do, nevertheless, regret that it seems reactionary. I believe the day may come when it will sound reactionary to oppose euthanasia and abortion, as it has already become reactionary to oppose divorce and artificial birth prevention. I further foresee the possibility under a State medical service, of doctors being compelled to procure abortions and kill the unfit. If artificial insemination shall have been accepted in that day, it will undoubtedly be considered reactionary for a man to refuse to allow his wife to receive the treatment.

In the modern state, what is permissible in one generation easily becomes compulsory in the next. If not likely, it is at least not impossible that artificial insemination may tomorrow be thought morally sound and socially smart. The day after tomorrow it may be imposed upon the wives of the poor, who, for one reason or other, have been unable to produce children. It is for these and kindred reasons that the Catholic theologian has not felt called upon to give lengthy consideration to this problem. There can be little doubt that the Catholic instinct is strong and constant in condemnation of the artificial insemination under review to-day. Except in the unlikely event of a reputable Catholic theologian questioning the instinctive Catholic recoil from this practice, it is unlikely that the Church will need to make any pronouncement further to the unvarnished condemnation of 1897.

Question and Answer

Q. Has the speaker never met a husband who loves his wife so much that he would rather father a child which has half of his own personality than a completely alien child ?

A. I think that is rather begging the question. Is it showing greater love in a man for him to want his wife to be pregnant by another man, or should the man anxious to give his wife the joy of a child, agree to adopt one ? I have never met a Catholic woman who wanted to be inseminated nor anyone who wanted his wife to have a child by another man.

VI. MEDICAL

By Dr. Mary Barton

This work has been a portion of my daily practice for about five years and I would emphasise that I think that in these matters personal experience must carry some weight. I must begin by giving the reasons why we ever started this work and I am going to commence with a few figures. As Mr. Walker has said, it is difficult to present precise figures at this stage, but about 10 per cent. of all marriages in this country, and probably in America, are sterile. In our own cases—the figure is several thousand—in about 60 per cent. of the infertile marriages the male partner is affected. In about 3 per cent. of marriages the male partner is hopelessly sterile. In those cases in which all has been done that can be done we are left with this picture—a marriage which has been, perhaps, happy in a way up to that time except for the increased longing of the wife for a child. There has been a good home with everything complete except that there is no child, but now something else enters into it. After consulting a specialist the wife knows herself to be fertile as far as science can assume these things and she knows that her husband is sterile. I can assure you that there is no more disruptive element which can enter into married life than this business of a fertile woman living with a man whom she knows can never give her a child.

It seems to me that in some way it destroys the basis of the relationship. For many years before we took up this particular solution we watched many a marriage go to pieces on these grounds. There is no stronger urge in the developed woman, in my experience, than that of bearing children, to experience maternity and to have a child from her own body. Adoption, therefore, even if enough children could be provided to go round, would not meet the case. None of us would suggest that adultery is the answer and by that I mean adultery in the ordinarily accepted sense. It is true that Christian virtue may be sufficient. The woman may be able to overcome the difficulty. The couple may say that this is what God has decreed and they submit to it and make their lives in some other way. But for most of them that is a supremely difficult thing to do. In my experience many who have had very great moral strength have become peculiar against their will. They have found themselves unbalanced, resentful and frustrated, and for that reason have been very much less good wives than they would have been otherwise. It seems to me that women can put up with almost anything in life except being denied the experience of maternity. I cannot, of course, generalise to such an extent as to say that there is no woman for whom adoption is not the solution. Sometimes adoption can be the solution but in medical experience and in that of others it does not solve 70 per cent. of the cases.

We could tell these people to go away and sublimate this urge, to do something else. Maybe we shall come to the conclusion ultimately that that is the proper thing to do. I can only say that my heart is not hard enough. I know personally, having children of my own, what the having and bearing and rearing of children means, and I could not say to a woman who came to me in an agony of distress and longing that I must reject her plea. For that reason my colleagues and I have taken up this solution. I believe most firmly in family life. I do not think that in most cases the relationship between men and women can develop to the full without sharing in the care and upbringing of children. I agree with Professor James that the family is the nucleus of society, but I cannot see how the father is eliminated from the home and the family. I cannot see how it can be said that the primary relationship between husband and wife is destroyed. In our experience it is nothing of the sort. You have to think of the effect on the woman of the extreme generosity and understanding of a husband who is not willing to force his wife to suffer from the results of his own disability. Furthermore, the husband remains the husband. He is the man who brings the child up, and it is his child to all intents and purposes. He remains her husband, her support and her companion, and in no sense is the structure of the marriage altered.

To those critics who have attacked us and who have suggested that we do this for lucrative purposes I would point out that it is far easier for us to refuse to do it. No doctor really likes playing with unsafe material. This is a question which is still under consideration and we have had a great deal of criticism for what we have done. It would have been much easier for us not to do it and, so far as the question of gain is concerned, it would be much more lucrative to treat hopelessly infertile, or almost infertile, people for long periods of time knowing full well that there was no hope of their recovery. Who are the people who ask for this treatment ? In five years I, personally, have had only two requests from unmarried women. I do not need to tell you that I did not grant their request. I have had people come to me who were in all walks of life and from every denomination. Although we do exercise the right to refuse couples who do not seem to us to be the right kind, we have only had to refuse on very rare occasions. Mostly the people are eminently deserving of this assistance according to our standards ; they are people who have every conceivable right to want to bring up children.

We have also been criticised for daring to make some choice in this matter. It seems to me that if we are going to take any responsibility at all—and we do feel a very great sense of responsibility—it is very important that we should do all we can to safeguard the future of children who come into these homes. We never persuade anybody; in fact, if there seems to be the slightest reason for dissuading people we do so. I cannot see that a doctor would persuade anyone against their own sense of rightness to do such a thing.

What is our usual procedure? Firstly, we make quite sure of the medical grounds for arranging for a donor. We make as reasonably sure as we can that the marriage is suitable, that the couple are happy together and that they have good reason to want to continue to remain together. We explain the legal implications and we insist that the matter should remain a secret. We have to do that to avoid the complication that the most appalling damage might be done to a little child by the discovery that his father was not, in fact, his father. If this is going to be done at all, I think the child should never know. The child should be born as the child of the man concerned and should be brought up to believe that that man is its father. We make a great point of obtaining written consent because we have to guard against one partner saying that he or she has gone behind the other's back. We test the fertility of the wife and then comes the question of the donor. In this country the work is small. In five years we have had only about 300 children conceived by this means. We do not have donors on anything like the scale arranged in America. Our practice is to find donors—an extremely difficult job—from the ranks of married men with families because we wish to have people with strong family desires, men whose parental instinct is satisfied and we want to see the progeny as well as know about the past generation. We have made a point of intelligence and we have also made a point of these men being good men.

To become a donor is not a pleasure. It is extremely difficult to obtain such a service from anybody in this country. We give as much information as we can to the couple but we never allow the donor to know precisely to whom the material goes, nor does he know if it is successful. We found that it was much better that he should not. Although this entails great trust, either you trust your doctor or you do not. To my mind there is no difference in this situation from the position of the surgeon or the obstetrician. Either you trust them or you do not and maybe you will think it wiser not to. Again, we never use donation where there can be any question of the husband not living with his wife ; we could not allow anyone to be in a position to prove adultery against the wife.

I should like to add that amongst these children, all of whom were healthy children, we had only two minor abnormalities, one a hernia and the other a single undescended testicle. The children have been happy and have been very much appreciated. I know that a grateful letter proves nothing but I think that to read one will be of interest. The husband of the writer of the letter was a young airman. After about two years—they were married at the beginning of the war—during part of which time they were separated, he was brought down in an air crash and his genital apparatus was completely smashed up. The couple came to me for attention and I arranged donation. The letter says : " This is to tell you how very much my husband and I appreciate the wonderful help and kindness which you have given us and we hope you will be able to give us some help again. . . . We are both thrilled about the coming event and my husband says he finds it hard to believe that it is not his own child. He seems as excited as I am about it, for you have solved what seemed to be a hopeless situation and what would have resulted in an unhappy, childless marriage. Please do not hesitate to use this letter should it be necessary. . . ."

I had a very similar case where a young man of Jewish origin was brutally kicked in his vital parts in one of the Mosley demonstrations and thereby lost his right to have children. I am not a pioneer and although it is very difficult for me not to appear so, I should like to say definitely that it would not make much difference to me if the whole affair were made illegal or was shown to be wrong by the Church. I cannot see that in any circumstances it could become a widespread practice because it seems to me that it is essentially something which meets individual needs here and there, and, secondly, it seems to me that secrecy is essential to its success. I cannot conceive of a couple turning up at a clinic for A.I.D. where their details would be taken by a clinical assistant, typed by a clerk, read by the nurse and carried by the out-patient porter into the doctor's consulting room and so forth. I do not believe that any of these people who come and ask for these services would consider it if it were done through our hospitals. I feel that this is essentially a moral question. I respect the attitude of the Roman Catholic Church in this matter and I think we should regard it as something which is not inevitably progress. The greatest problem of our time is the battle between science and ethics and I am the last person who would be willing to place myself unequivocably and irrevocably on the side of science.

Questions and Answers

Q. Were the cases which Dr. Barton mentioned donor cases or was there artificial insemination from the husband ? What preparations are made beforehand in relation to probable malformation of the infant ? Because a husband is proved sterile, will artificial insemination solve the problem ? The wife remains tied to a man whom she apparently finds distasteful and inadequate at least subconsciously. Otherwise she would not seek elsewhere to have her own body satisfied. Is it not an indictment against women to say that because a wife finds her husband sterile she must do something about it, whereas it is taken for granted that if a husband is told his wife is sterile he is considered very brutal if he does not think of her with even greater affection than before ?

A. I was referring to A.I.D. If I had been speaking of A.I.H. there would have been thousands of cases from which to quote. With regard to malformation, it is impossible to provide against an occasional abnormality but with this method there is probably a lower percentage than in ordinary marriage. There is highly fecund and satisfactory stock on one side but we shall have to have more cases before we can tell whether the abnormality rate is actually lower. The risk of the couple having a child with an abnormality is present as in ordinary marriage ; we have no means of protecting anybody against that risk. I cannot see that you can say that the woman inevitably dislikes her husband in these cases. In most cases where dislike occurs it is after some years when the husband has denied his wife the chance of becoming pregnant. Where the difficulty has been met by A.I.D. I have never seen the relationship turn to dislike. I have never yet found the father who did not love the child. The father forgets the origin of the child and in some odd way he notices things about a baby which remind him of things in his own childhood. It occurs to him that it is just possible that it might be his own child. I do not see that the question of the fecund husband and the sterile wife enters into this at all.

Q. Dr. Barton referred to her colleagues. Is there a clinic for this work ?

A. I mentioned my private colleagues. There are no recognised public clinics in England for this work.

Q. If the consent of the wife and husband is required in the case of A.I.D., is the consent of the donor's wife required so far as the donation of the semen is concerned ?

A. Of course. Otherwise there might be a risk of the donor being accused of adultery, although I do not see how it could be found out. These donors do it with the full understanding, acquiescence and support of their wives.

Q. Dr. Barton has said that there is no danger of a clinic being opened for this purpose as people would be ashamed to have all the details of their case known. Are they likely to be more ashamed of artificial insemination than of V.D. ?

A. I do not know if the questioner knows the extreme secrecy with which matters are conducted in V.D. hospitals. I never said that clinics might not be established because in this age anything might happen, but from my personal point of view I think they would defeat their own object.

VII. THEOLOGICAL
(The Church of England)

By Rev. G. L. Russell, M.B., Ch.B.

I ought to say at once that I cannot claim, for the opinions on this subject which I shall be expressing, any authority but my own. No official statement has yet been made on behalf of the Church of England. There is now at work upon a full enquiry into artificial insemination a Commission of theologians, doctors, lawyers, psychologists and others, appointed by the Archbishop of Canterbury, which will in due course report to him. Whether the findings of that Commission will later be published by authority, and whether they will form the basis of any official pronouncement from Lambeth, I have not the least idea. In the meanwhile, an Anglican can do no more than voice his own opinion, in the light of his Christian Faith and the best information and evidence now available.

It is next to impossible for an Anglican considering such a matter as this, and at this particular time, not to invoke, in doing so, the whole conception of the Natural Law. If artificial insemination (whether homologous, or heterologous, or both) is wrong, then it is wrong not simply for Christians but for everybody. If it is wrong, it is so because if offends against the nature of man as man, of marriage as marriage, of the family as the basic *natural* unit of human society.

Natural Law (if I may adapt one of the simpler definitions of it) is the ordered structure of the world and of human behaviour in it, constituted by the Divine Reason, and therefore the standard by which the activities of all creatures ought to be regulated and must be judged. Much in the universe behaves (so far as we can tell) as it was made and meant to behave.

Stars and sulphuric acid, moles and molecules, appear to be controlled by a law of their own being which (if they were rational creatures) we should say they "perfectly" obeyed. It is true that in the plant and animal world there is some evidence of spontaneous and aberrant development, of which science can at present say no more than that "it happens." Nevertheless, it is only in men and women and the life of human society, that the gap between what IS and what OUGHT TO BE reaches notable proportions, and raises the problems with which philosophers and moralists have always been concerned. It would be hard indeed to find anyone who did not admit this distinction, in some form at least, between IS and OUGHT. It is assumed as axiomatic, in virtually all discussion, that men and women do not, or do not always, behave as they *might* behave. There is for all of them at least the possibility however remote, however qualified, of *different* behaviour from that which they normally exhibit. It is usually implied that this different behaviour would somehow also be *better*—whatever criteria are used for assessing the *better*. (You will observe that I assume—there is no time to argue the case—that rigid and orthodox behaviourism is not really a tenable philosophy !)

The Law is called "natural" not in contrast with "supernatural" but in contrast with positive human law—the legal statutes and codes which should be framed and are to be judged by reference to Natural Law. This—the "Law of Nature" as it is often called, especially when applied to human behaviour—is neither fully clear nor wholly obscured for men and women in their unredeemed condition. In them, "the understanding is darkened," so that it is not always possible for them to discern—or discern fully—what is their natural behaviour, still less to follow it. And this obscurity, and uncertainty, may be greater (in relation to one particular field of action) at one period than at another. For example, it is harder today for non-Christian men (and harder even for Christians) to see what is *natural* for them through the whole range of relationships between the sexes, than it was for men who lived 100, or 1000, years ago. That is to imply *not* that people's actual behaviour is better or worse *now* than it was at some time in the past: only that it is harder for them now than it was then to be sure how they *ought* to behave—at least in some parts of their lives. The Church believes and teaches that it is *natural* (in the full sense of the word which I have been using) for a man to be joined, in marriage, to one woman, for life, to the exclusion of all others. But no-one will deny that the circumstances of contemporary Western society, and still more the ideas and assumptions which govern most men and women who live in it, make it more difficult for those who are not instructed Christians to accept that view as simply *the truth*—something proceeding from the real nature of man as well as the nature of marriage—as the only terms upon which it is possible to know *what marriage is.*

The two-fold effect of the Christian Revelation upon those who receive it is (i) to illuminate for them what natural behaviour is, and (ii) to make it possible for them to follow it. Then, it may be said, what is the use of talking about the Natural Law to people who are not Christian? The answer is this. Even non-Christian men may discern, in varying measure, how they *ought* to behave. That they *do not* behave like that, and know that they *cannot*, is the first and necessary step towards accepting the Christian Faith. But the essential point is that *all* men have, written into their reason, some capacity at least to know what they should do. Some part at least of that true meaning of life which shines in the Person of Christ, shines faintly in the most brutish man.

Secondly, the pattern of human behaviour which is called " natural " is not prescribed only for Christians. For them it becomes, in a way not true for others, possible of realisation. But it is not that this pattern is offered to Christians and not to others. There is only one truly human life for all men everywhere. In and for Christians the vital impulse of supernature—what the Church calls *grace*—can bring that life to perfection. But the rest of mankind is not simply doomed to utter chaos and unrelieved frustration. Apart from the possibility of the fulfilment of the natural, there remain possibilities of retaining, and affirming, the minimum requirements for social order, for human justice and freedom. They are not enough —if they were, where were the need for redemption ? But human life built on these basic sanctions and securities is so much more tolerable and significant, than it can ever be without them, that it is a *Christian* concern to maintain and strengthen them against all that threatens their destruction.

The Church vis-a-vis the world is in a position not unlike that of a doctor whose patient has diabetes. It is the doctor's duty to tell the patient that what his system lacks is *insulin* : only a new supply of insulin can restore him to health. But suppose the patient to be averse to insulin : he does not believe in it, and will have none of it. Then the doctor is bound to tell him that while insulin is the only *remedy* for his condition, there are other measures he can take which may alleviate it, or at least prevent it from deteriorating further. He must go on a diet and regulate his life in this way and that. To be sure, he cannot expect, by adopting these substitute measures to live the full, free and " normal " life which insulin would secure for him. But these may at least keep him going, and prevent a complete breakdown.

So with the souls and societies of men. Not any re-arrangement, or new adjustment, of the elements already present in the human situation, can bring mankind salvation—but only some force and power coming in from outside it. Still, apart from this, and on another level than that of grace, it can be made more easy or more difficult, more seemingly " normal " or more " odd," for men and women to do the things that express, and do not frustrate, their human nature. There are real, though often fine, distinctions between those actions and customs which do violence to the natural pattern, and those which do not.

In complete harmony with this conception of Natural Law, and indeed required by it, is the notion of Christian morality as a pursuit of ENDS rather than mere conformity to a rule of conduct. In every situation demanding action, what will ultimately determine the nature of the action—if it is to be the proper response to that situation—is reference to the purpose of human life, the nature and destiny of human beings. " What am I ? What am I for ? " These are the ultimate questions affecting conduct—which could be defined as a choice of *means* to the chosen *end*. There is, of course, a multiplicity of *intermediate* ends, related to some immediate, particular, action. To treat myopia, to enable a man to see better, so that he may do his work, in order to support his family, and fulfil his vocation as husband and father—these are simple examples. The test of the " rightness " or " wrongness " of each limited end or objective is whether or no it serves the *final* end--the goal of existence, the ultimate good for Man. Thus the questions we have to ask about this or that procedure in Artificial Insemination are all concerned with the *true ends* of sexual activity, of marriage, of family life.

It is obvious, I imagine, that there is a quite definite distinction between homologous and heterologous insemination. The first is no more than the attempt—by whatever means—to secure the fulfilment of one of those three "causes" for which matrimony was ordained. No-one disputes that : the only difference of opinion is about the method used. As Fr. Henry Davis has said : " It is not immoral for human seed which has been ejected in the effort of intercourse to be put at the mouth of the vagina " (or elsewhere) " and for the doctor or nurse then to make sure of its entry by artificial methods." The obtaining of seed by masturbation has been condemned. It is obvious that in a majority of cases where masturbation is resorted to, it might be avoided—by the substitution of some attempt at least at normal intercourse and the collection of semen thereafter. But if there were, for the insemination of a wife with her husband's semen, no practicable alternative to masturbation, I do not myself believe that on moral grounds this course should be prohibited. For in this case the act, being directed towards the completion (*ex hypothesi* impossible without it) of the procreative end of the marriage, loses its character of self-abuse. I cannot bring myself to believe that it could ever be God's will that a married couple should remain childless *merely* because one act of this kind is required to promote conception.

The consideration of A.I.D. raises questions of an entirely different kind. The fundamental one is, of course, whether or not it constitutes adultery. I understand that, so far as the Law of England is concerned, there is no doubt on this point. A.I.D. involves adultery, whatever the motives, circumstances, or consequences. In this the Law reflects not only the traditional view of marriage, but ordinary common sense. The ordinary man or woman, knowing that Mrs. X had given birth to a child in London while her husband had been in New York for the previous year (I exclude, of course, A.I.H.) will hardly need the expert advice of lawyers before coming to an opinion. A wife might, as has been pointed out, be producing children all over the world without her husband's assistance ; and is she to claim that she has faithfully and punctiliously fulfilled her marriage vows ?

It will be said that some married women, who have never been pregnant, have an inordinate desire for children, and will never be happy without them. The moral question here is whether such a desire—one which leads a wife to demand a child as a result of her fertilisation with alien seed—is, in strict truth *inordinate* : one which exceeds the proper bounds of desire. There are some whose sexual impulses might be similarly described : but that is no defence in a court of Law. They are required to control their desires, however imperious. On what rational ground are we to say that while *sexual* desires ought not to be indulged at will, *parental* desires may be ? The plight of the childless wife should call out our deepest sympathy. But I could not myself stretch sympathy to include the condoning of what I am clear must be called adultery.

Further, A.I.D. involves an unnatural separation of the unitive and procreative ends of marriage. This might be held to apply as much to A.I.H. as to A.I.D. ; and in certain circumstances this would, I think, be true.

We know too little as yet of the psychological relationship between sexual impotence and the emotional capacity for parenthood. And until we know more I think we should hesitate to say that in *all* cases of impotence in the husband, A.I.H. should be advised. Nevertheless, even where the sex act cannot be properly performed, there is between husband and wife (at least potentially) a whole range of personal intercourse, contact, and union which are *ex hypothesi* ruled out in the case of A.I.D.

I have heard the argument that for those who are ready to allow the intentional separation of intercourse from its procreative end which contraception makes possible, there can be no logical objection to the process reversed—i.e. to procreation apart from intercourse. I think the analogy is false. The separation of ends involved in contraception is justified (if at all) because it allows *one* of them—the unitive—to be fulfilled in circumstances which must otherwise (i.e. apart from contraception) frustrate *both* ends of marriage, by the cessation of all marital intercourse. A.I.D., on the other hand, does not serve either union or procreation *within the marriage*. Husband and wife are not, as a result of it, united (sexually), nor is the procreative end of *their marriage* furthered, since what is substituted for it is procreation of the wife and a man who is not her husband.

There is a further wound in the natural pattern inflicted by A.I.D. It substitutes for the family, which is the community of parents and *the children begotten by them*, a group of persons differently related. To say that as a result of illegitimacy and adoption this is a process continually going on, is to evade the real issue. The adopted child *may* be brought up in ignorance of his true parentage : but the State insists that anyone has the right to discover, if they wish, what are the facts of the case. That is the significance of the Adoption Register. As for illegitimacy, no-one seriously regards it as a *solution* of any problem. I say nothing of the perjury involved in the false declaration to the Registrar; but the fraud which is practised both upon child and community in withholding from both knowledge as to his true identity to which each is entitled, seems a more serious matter. A child has a right, universally conceded, not only to two parents, but to the *knowledge of them*. The position of boys and girls, and men and women, who have not the faintest notion who were their fathers, and no means of finding out, is not conducive to mental and spiritual health.

To sum up:—If we ask, of A.I.D., whether it may fulfil, or whether it must frustrate, the ends or purposes for which marriage exists, answers seem to be these. It does not fulfil the procreative end, which (*ex hypothesi*) is already stultified. A.I.D. does not revive it; it substitutes for it something else altogether—the procreation of a wife and a man who is not her husband. The *sexual* relationship of marriage is not *directly* affected by A.I.D., but only by its results. Child-bearing may conceivably affect it physically, maternity psychologically—though this latter properly belongs to the third aspect of marriage, " the society help and comfort which the one ought to have of the other." Here, the psychological evidence is of paramount importance, and unfortunately there is so far not a great deal of it. It is argued that as a result of the presence of the child conceived by A.I.D., both husband and wife may be happier and their relationship cemented. I think that we should all agree that in some cases anyway this may be so. It is, however, quite obvious that there is risk of the relationship being later on impaired—by jealousy, inferiority feelings, and so forth. But there is also this to be said. Suppose it the case that A.I.D. could in general, or in a particular instance, add to the personal harmony and even the sexual satisfaction of husband and wife—i.e. suppose *two* ends of the marriage served by defeating the third. Precisely the same might be said of adultery, in the common sense of that term. It is conceivable (I have known it happen) that a wife, or husband, may learn from a lover what later—after a written reconciliation between the two spouses, or even without it—makes for the sexual and personal enrichment of the marriage. I say that is at any rate conceivable. But is anyone rash enough to assert that because, in certain circumstances, such is the result of adultery, it is legitimate for any husband to take a mistress or any wife a lover? Some people, I know, are prepared to argue for that. But even they would hardly do so on the ground that *Christian marriage* was what they contended for, and wished to safeguard—but rather the right to sexual experience outside marriage, and so forth. And I submit that it is no more illogical to claim to support *marriage* by permitting ordinary adultery, that to claim to support it by promoting A.I.D. I need hardly say that I intend no kind of slur upon those who plead for it—I am sure they want, as much as any of us, to see happy, successful, and enduring marriages. But I think they are mistaken in their view of what marriage *is*, and of the conditions which are required for it, and of those which must violate its essential structure. Not all, but most, of the disagreements which vex our world today are not about ends, but means. And I think this is one of them.

VIII. LEGAL

By Mr. J. P. Ashworth

I am going to take up your time for a few moments considering some of the legal aspects of this subject and it is only fair to say at the start, and it is probably within your knowledge, that there has been no study by the Courts of this country of artificial insemination as such. So far as one can deal with the question at all from the legal aspect one must consider what problems would arise and what kind of principles would be applied if the law were to stand as it stands to-day. I would only add to that that if artificial insemination were to be common or widespread, I think you will agree that some form of legislation would be required and therefore different principles might be enacted in dealing with it. The first problem which arises is the question of the doctor who administers. He is not at the moment committing any offence against the law unless the consent which is given is not genuine. This question of consent is, to my mind, something very much deeper than one which is merely answered by saying, "We obtained a signed statement." The cases which so far appear to have arisen have been in some measure successful cases but the law, as you know, tends to deal with failures.

It is the failures which would give rise to this question of consent in a very acute form from the doctor's point of view. The woman might well change her mind, and if all that a doctor has to safeguard him is a certificate, possibly signed by both, one can visualise difficult and distasteful issues coming before the tribunal as to the measure of consent. Apart from consent, the crime of rape, or, if not that, of something very close to it, is concerned. The alternative would be to get some higher form of consent, something, for example, on oath. I foresee great difficulty in that from the parents' point of view because one can imagine from what Dr. Barton has said, that secrecy has to be preserved if possible at all costs and there would be a natural reluctance on the part of any woman and any husband to go before a Commissioner of Oaths and make a statutory declaration that there was consent to what had to be done. You have got to weigh in the balance, from the doctor's point of view, what may be a worthless piece of paper and, on the other hand, a document which the parents may be unwilling to sign.

Assuming that consent has been obtained, the next difficulty arises in regard to registration. I do not know what is done because I have no experience in the matter, but I have no hesitation in saying that if A.I.D. is used, and the mother registers her husband as the father, she is making a false statement under the Perjury Act. The penalty is a maximum of £50 if the matter is dealt with summarily and it can be worse if it is dealt with by indictment. The fact is, that she is committing an offence and so is her husband. I do not know what is done but it is an extremely difficult situation. You are met either with the requirement that you must commit an offence, or, as Dr. Barton has said, the very thing which is to be avoided and that is to proclaim to the world that the child is fatherless. A birth certificate will be required many times in one's life and either the information is not embodied in the column relating to the father or it contains a falsehood. I do not see any escape from that as the law stands at the moment and it is a problem which must come up in an acute form.

To go further, we will suppose that the child is born and that the difficulty of registration has been overcome. The next problem which would require very careful thought, and one which might arise in many cases, is the question of whether the child is legitimate or not, and as to that, I would say with little hesitation that it is illegitimate. You are bringing into the world a bastard ; let us face it. For good or ill, that is what is being done. The Russell case laid down in plain terms that fecundation *ab extra* that is, from without, is adultery and that the issue of such fecundation is illegitimate. Consider where that takes you. You may have a husband and wife interested in their own marriage settlement and in their uncle's will. It does not take much imagination to see scores of cases in which some property is left to these parents and to their issue. The *prima facie* ruling is that issue means legitimate issue. Let us see where that takes you. First of all, there may be third parties involved. It may be the issue of John Smith and his wife, or, in default of his wife, Joan Johnson. She is clearly interested in the situation which arises if there is no lawful issue. How are you going to meet that ? I understand that it is proposed in one quarter that one method would be to obtain an assurance from the parents at the time of insemination that there is no third party interested who may be overridden. I suggest that an assurance of that kind is not worth the paper it is written upon. How can the intentions of third parties, possibly unknown to them at the time, be known ? The husband and wife do not know the terms of the wills of the various relatives, if such a will exists. Even if they were in the fortunate position of knowing what had already been put on paper by deposition or otherwise, there is nothing to stop anyone, from the moment they have given the assurance, from leaving them money on those terms. So an assurance of that sort, comforting as it may be to the doctor, is really not worth anything at all. You cannot protect the interests of a child that may come from artificial insemination against the claims of third parties.

The Russell case, which you can no doubt remember, happened 22 years ago and is the most famous, recent authority for a rule of English law which there has been for 200 years or more, namely, that a husband or a wife is not permitted to give evidence in a court of law to the effect that he or she has not had intercourse with the other for the purpose of bastardizing the child. In the Russell case you will remember, that the wife had a child and the husband sought to give evidence to the effect that he had not had intercourse with her, and it was rejected. That rule, as I see it, has got to be kept very closely in mind in consideration of any legal problems on this topic. It is not so much a question of what applies at the time; it is what happens afterwards. One is liable to think of these topics merely from the point of view that all will go well. I did not know, but I understand from Dr. Barton, that there have been no failures, but that will not happen always and what one has to consider as a lawyer is the situation supposing that husband and wife fall out. It may be that the woman will regret the experience she has gone through; one has heard of such cases. Or the husband may regret giving consent.

But whatever the cause, what will happen when they do fall out? I say frankly that the problems of the maintenance and custody of the child raise acute legal problems. The position is extremely difficult because there is this extraordinary situation. The husband and wife know themselves that the child which nominally bears their name and was born to the mother is not theirs, but neither of them can give evidence to bastardize the issue. Yet there is the fact, provable by the doctor, that in fact the child belongs to someone else. The mother will carry with her the duty of maintaining the child. She may share that with her husband, or not, but the question of whether he should not be allowed to say that he could not be the father raises a very difficult problem.

What can be said as to custody ? The mother has a claim to custody, but it has been laid down over and over again that the paramount consideration in these matters is the welfare of the child. What are you going to do in a case of that kind ? I am only pointing to these things as problems which may arise and I do not pretend to have the answer. What I am endeavouring to suggest is that any light-hearted assumption that having squared your morals about it the rest is easy is quite wrong.

I also understand that one method of practising artificial insemination is by mixing the semen of the donor with that of the husband. It is a device which to my mind at any rate certainly deserves the title of " artificial " and I cannot help thinking that, if it was sought to get round the illegitimacy of the child by that method, the Courts might be somewhat slow to show any sympathy towards it. None the less, it may be an answer to some of the things I have been putting to you, that in fact there is no proof that the child is A.I.D. in the fullest sense of the word, that is, an unknown father's child, but is possibly that and possibly the father's. That may be a way out, but if I may speak freely it is a way from which I should revolt.

Possibly it is not a very likely occurrence, but supposing the donor became known. We have been told that something like 50 inseminations might take place from one donor. The laws of chance are widespread, but the possibility of inter-marriage between the issue has already been mentioned from one point of view. I would only hold it out to you as a plain case of incest. If it were proved, involuntary although it might be, the fact would remain that an incestuous union had taken place. I am not talking of the question of penalty. The two parties would be most unlikely to know that they had shared their father, but, none the less, the fact would be there.

I hope I have said enough to show that there are difficult legal problems involved in this subject. If, as I said before, it became widespread, it is a matter which would have to be dealt with not by the existing law but by Parliament making a new law.

IX. MEDICAL

By Dr. Joan Malleson

UNTIL Dr. Mary Barton spoke, it seemed to me that this discussion lacked the point of view of the woman, which, after all, is a real one in such a debate. I am frequently surprised at the different way in which women respond to this subject as compared with men. Men often seem to forget the extraordinary depths of longing for a child which women will occasionally maintain even in the face of every obstacle. It is commonly accepted that women value child-bearing, but people without clinical experience tend to forget the case of the exceptional woman, to whom life seems absolutely nothing unless she can fulfil herself in that way. Such a woman does not necessarily marry for sexual union; she marries for a child and nothing in the world seems any good to her except a child. Such women can be encouraged to sublimate that desire by taking care of other people's children, but to some that suggestion is quite ridiculous. To offer motherhood " by proxy " to a woman of that kind is very much like offering a wife by proxy to a celibate man! Not all people can get their deepest emotional feelings satisfied by watching other people get what they themselves desire. When the husband of such a woman is sterile, she frequently fears that bitterness will creep into her marriage, particularly as the years advance: and this fear is expressed often by the husband, too. It is motives such as this which sometimes cause some couples to seek the help of donated insemination.

I find myself also thinking in this discussion that it is strange in a debate between lay people and the clergy that I, as a lay woman, seem to believe a little more in "goodness" than do the clergy! It has seemed to me from my experience that husbands and wives are *more* loving and generous than the clergy seem to find! I asked the Catholic speaker earlier in discussion whether he had ever found a husband who loved his wife so much that he would prefer a child which was hers to an adopted one alien to both of them. He replied that he had not; but I assure him they are not uncommon. I have been repeatedly impressed to find that among the finest and most loving type of husband this sort of generosity is not infrequently encountered. Indeed, it is only from such people that these requests are likely to come; for the couple must also have stability and courage to embark on such an undertaking.

For my part, I should feel that if the Churches closed their doors to such a couple who sought an inseminated child, that it would reveal a failure to comprehend much that is fine and good, and a callousness in dealing with one of life's deepest misfortunes. I do not believe that the Churches profit by forbidding acts which men and women may feel are morally and socially good. I see frequently the conflict caused to Roman Catholic couples over the matter of contraception; and when they feel impelled, as an alternative to lifelong celibacy, to adopt contraception in spite of their Church's teaching, I do not think it does good either for the individual or for the Church.

There may be some parallels to be drawn over Society's attitude to contraception and to this matter of artificial insemination. During twenty-five years, the viewpoint of most clergy to the matter of contraception has changed greatly; and, recalling this, is it not possible that they would be wise not to adjudicate finally on this other problem?

Although in a discussion of this sort one might think that there were a bevy of doctors urging such treatment to countless couples, in fact the number of sterility cases which could ever be considered suitable for such treatment would always be exceedingly small: only a small minority of cases are ineligible for any other treatment, and a much smaller number would be emotionally suitable for artificial insemination.

I would, therefore, put in a plea for the Churches not to forget that for a very few of their flock "goodness" in life may lie in this direction: and that to condemn such an action as unworthy may display a lack of vision which will later be regretted.

Questions and Answers

Q. Reference has been made to the mixing of the semen of the husband and of the donor. Can the speaker say what will be the result of that on the outlook of the husband in the marriage?

A. If the husband has had sexual intercourse with his wife during the month in which the artificial insemination took place, I have taken it for granted that one could never prove that the child was not his. Under the paternity laws it is maintained that if a husband and a lover have access to a woman in the same month the child is assumed to be legitimate.

X. MEDICAL

By J. V. O'Sullivan, M.D., F.R.C.S., F.R.C.O.G.

I should like to draw attention to a few points which I think would help in this discussion. In 1866 J. Marion Sims, one of the greatest gynæcologists, practised artificial insemination and heralded it as a great success. Later in his life he condemned it absolutely as an immoral medical practice.

Up to 1934, only 123 cases of artificial insemination in human beings could be found in the literature of the world. Schultze made 102 attempts with 12 successes. In 1928 Englemann went over the whole world literature and found 185 cases with 65 successes. Between 1928 and 1941 Cohen, Goldberg, Schatz, Israel and Englemann published several reports. At the end of 1941 two lady doctors in America reported the number of cases in America to be 9,489 successful pregnancies, showing the rapidity with which artificial insemination had increased. This increase is noteworthy. Their results were analysed by the American Gynæcological Society whose conclusion was that the figures of these two ladies did not stand analysis, showing, in other words, that the extraordinary successes they claimed were invalid. They claimed that all the babies were perfect, which is, of course, impossible.

You have already heard observations as to the methods used. I think it is generally agreed, that apart from using the masturbation method everything should be done to get the wife impregnated with the husband's semen. One speaker has pointed out that masturbation for the purpose of procreation would do no harm, but that is not always so because one has to consider the effect of masturbation on the donor from a psychological and general point of view.

Lastly we come to a serious problem in artificial insemination, namely, the choice of donor. The religious background, education, race, character and so forth have to be considered in association with the prospective mother and father. You can see how difficult it is. In some cases in America they have to hire students as donors and pay them five dollars per specimen, because it is impossible to get any other donors.

Next we come to the legal aspect and here is a small point I should like to make. A case of adultery was sustained in the supreme court of Ontario in 1921 where donor semen was used in artificial insemination. The next question is that of secrecy, and we are told that secrecy is vital. Most of us will agree that the basic unit of society is the family, and a happy wife, normally fertile, is quite a different being in the eyes of her friends and neighbours, to a woman artificially inseminated. If a large number of babies were born from a limited number of donors it is obvious that some of the children may meet and intermarry. There lies a danger. The necessity for permanent silence must also be a lifelong strain on the father and mother and may react on the children.

I feel that before we get to the stage of practising artificial insemination a great deal more work should be done on the medical side. I quite agree that where there is no sperm at all there is little hope. Still there may be some surgical method whereby such people can be rendered potent. I know in America they claim some success in this sphere.

Lastly, I emphasize that we, as physicians, should devote more time to fundamental research in fertility. I am sure we doctors will be rewarded with findings which will obviate the use of donor semen, if not eradicate it altogether. Surely our duty to our patients is the wider use of preventive medicine and reparation rather than substitution.

XI. THEOLOGICAL
(The Free Churches)

BY THE REV. DR. T. G. DUNNING. M.A.

A RELIGIOUS ruling may rise from two sources. It may be given in an explicit injunction in the Word of God, or may be stated in an official pronouncement of the Christian Church. With regard to the former, we are not surprised that the Scripture contains no reference to artificial insemination. It was unknown when the Bible was written but nevertheless note should be taken of a custom to which frequent reference is made in the Old Testament and which bears on the subject of childless unions. I refer to the Levirate marriage custom. This enjoined that when a husband died childless, his younger brother took the widow and the issue of such union was counted the heir of the deceased husband and not of the actual father. The classic instance of this is the story of Tamar in the 38th Chapter of the Book of Genesis.

Of the many lands in which this custom was honoured and the various origins attributed to it, and the different purposes it was intended to serve, I need not speak here. Two observations alone will suffice. First, that this custom was so widespread and prevailed for so long and even acquired the sanction of religion, indicates how deep-seated was the compassion for the childless couple, a compassion reinforced now by Christian considerations. Nevertheless, this custom fell into abeyance and that it did so in spite of the support of tradition and law must be attributed mainly to the growth of the consciousness and claims of the individual as such, a consciousness and claims that have deep religious significance as we shall see later.

Turning from Scripture to the Church, I may say that

the Free Churches have delivered no pronouncement on this subject and it would need a greater optimism than I possess to anticipate that at some future date they will deliver a unanimous and final ruling on it. The Free Churches are somewhat divided over the issue of divorce and on such related questions as the remarriage of the divorced. A similar division of opinion can be detected with regard to human artificial insemination.

This statement will at least indicate where I stand. I speak at the request of the Free Churches but not on behalf of them. I speak only as a Free Churchman. Nevertheless, I intend to apply to this subject principles accepted by us all. The first is that there can be no religious objections against the artificial as such. Those who protest against the artificial should indicate what they mean by the natural. For instance, in this connection they would probably include in the natural such things as drugs and forceps, twilight sleep and Cæsarean methods. Moreover, these people would hardly deny to a soldier whose life blood was being shed for his country the benefit that could come through a transfusion of blood by artificial methods and we should recognise that there is no biological difference between artificial insemination and other substitute serums. That there is more than biology in this we shall recognise very clearly later. For the moment we are considering the religious significance of the artificial as such.

Moreover, the God who made nature and determined the natural processes also made the mind that comprehends nature and co-operates with her. The God who said "Be fruitful and multiply" also said: "Replenish the earth and subdue it," and its subjection will require the use of what is called the artificial. In fact, we may say that the understanding and use of nuclear energy has its legitimate place in that subjugation.

The atom is His and He made it, for His hands formed the dry land. It ought to be recognised that if we are really going to eliminate the artificial then the whole pharmacopœia and all the benefits of surgical skill must be relinquished. Moreover, we have to recognise what a wonderful handmaid of Christian compassion the so-called "artificial" may be. It is asserted that the feeding of the hungry and the clothing of the ill-clad will merit eternal recognition and gratitude. Yet the bread thus given may have been baked in a so-called artificial oven and the garment may have been woven in a so-called artificial mill. Should gratitude, therefore, be less spontaneous and deep if medical skill brings to the empty arms of the hitherto childless wife a babe that is both her own and her husband's? I can therefore see no ground whatever for religious objection to the artificial as such.

Secondly, it is the will of God that marriage should take place and that children should be produced. This does not imply that procreation is the inevitable issue of a union or that, when it does not result, any means to reach that end can be justified. God had in marriage purposes other than reproduction. Certainly the enrichment of the personalities involved is one of the first objectives. Nevertheless, one cannot but recognise what the Divine intention is, and whatever promotes the realisation of that, other things being equal, should have His blessing. When the Divine intention is not realised in the married union, we ought, therefore, to see not only how some substitute for the wanted child can be found—for example, by means of artificial insemination—but we ought also to labour strenuously to track down the causes of sterility and thus enable the united couple to have a child that is not half, but entirely their own. It is a profoundly impressive fact to recognise that twenty years ago so much attention was being given to contraception. To-day adequate conception is predominant in the minds of many and I welcome what has been said tonight about studying more deeply the causes of sterility and what remedies may be found for that.

In fact, we may look backward and ask whether some of the regrettable sterility to to-day is not due to what is already artificial in human life. I am merely speculating, but if that be so, we are only using the artificial to restore nature's proper balance.

So far, consideration has been given only to the effort to enable a husband and wife to have a child of their own. We now have to think of other uses of artificial insemination and one cannot feel that to these the sanction of religion can be given as in the former case. Nor can it be denied equally to all types. For convenience I shall classify them into two categories. First, those that must be entirely barred—for example, where a wife secures insemination by a donor simply to maintain the husband's esteem, or where an unmarried girl may secure insemination to compel a man to marry her, or even where an unmarried girl may wish artificial insemination so that she may have a child of her own. To bring life into this world simply to serve such secondary or such deceptive ends is undoubtedly wrong. We reach more of a borderline case where a husband and wife agree to insemination by an unknown donor. Before examining what has to be said against this, we should frankly admit what there is in its favour. The donor can be medically certified to be biologically fit for this task ; his identity can remain completely unknown to the couple involved. They may choose the kind of characteristics they want in their child. Moreover, I think there is not in this the unhealthy and illicit love-making that may be associated with contraception by an unmarried couple. I see a distinction there.

Nevertheless, there is much to be said against this and I intend to examine it in the light of another strong religious principle, the divine sanctity of the human personality. This has to be stressed to-day against many modern tendencies. For example, against the emphasis on the totalitarian State which may ignore or suppress individual significance and value, against the increasing social controls that may dry up individual initiative and responsibility, and against the increasing mechanisation of human life. Man is more than a political entity, an industrial cog and an economic unit. He is a child of God, of infinite value in his Father's eyes. In the light of this principle let us look at the individuals involved in artificial insemination.

We have first of all the donor. To serve the purposes of insemination he has, without love, to condition himself in a way in which he should never condition himself without love. He has thus to make himself responsible for offspring towards which he is under obligation to be indifferent for ever afterwards. This is against nature. It violates to some extent the sanctity of his personality. It is wrong to liken him, as some have done, to the nasty boy who masturbates. In fact, altruism may move the donor in his service, but taking this practice so far as it concerns him alone, one feels that it is not compatible with the sanctity of his personality.

Every child has the right to a good father and a good mother. Therefore, I feel that this rules out any sanction for the single girl receiving artificial insemination. Of course, I know that she may say that her nature demands that right, but as against that the child that would be the issue also has rights, particularly the right to a good father and a good mother. Further, it may be asserted that where a wife with the approval of her husband obtains artificial insemination by a donor, the husband intends, as well as the wife, to be a good parent to the child. If it were merely a biological matter it would be simple, but there is more than biology involved here. There are deep psychological, emotional and even spiritual implications.

Turning again to the child itself, we have to ask ourselves if the child of artificial insemination can ever be the same as the child of natural insemination. In other words—and here I welcome the knowledge of the expert—does not the mode of conception influence the product of conception ? There is in the loving embrace of a devoted husband and wife a rich emotional content that must surely be entirely absent from the use of the syringe and the test tube. The success of stud farm methods has no relevance whatever here because we are in depths far beyond biological ones.

With regard to the legal father, although the husband may in all sincerity give his consent to artificial insemination, can he be sure of his future emotions ? Can he be certain that he can think with equanimity of his wife fostering into human life the donation of an unknown man ? Moreover, if the child proves to be disappointing, or should friction arise between husband and wife, who can tell how detrimental to reconciliation may be the unusual origin of the child ? To simplify the issue, if medical skill at some future date could raise parthenogenesis to the human level the issue would be enormously simplified because the third person, or the second man, would be entirely eliminated. In fact, where the husband and wife so ardently desire a child why should they not follow the normal course of adoption ? For artificial insemination it can be said that the child is half theirs. That is true, but the other half has its own problems. Towards the adopted child, however, the husband and wife can feel that they have an equal relationship and this is not without its advantages.

With regard to the mother, it is asserted that the childless wife by means of artificial insemination may obtain the satisfying experience of pregnancy and the relief of grave nervous tensions. We need not dispute this, but on the ground of this alone much could also be said for a single girl resorting to artificial insemination. Disdaining adultery she might ask for artificial insemination so that she may have the satisfying experience and be relieved of certain tensions. In other words, it is questionable whether a child should be produced for these rather secondary ends. At any rate the single girl is so often advised to sublimate her sex instincts that one might ask also if this is too hard for the childless wife. One has to think of the wonderfully valuable service that has been rendered by childless couples who have given to some of the unwanted and the unloved childhood of our land the care and love they would have gladly lavished upon children of their own. One will never be able to measure what the nation owes to this splendid sublimation of a natural instinct. Apart from that, the question still has to be answered whether the mother, like the legal father, can be sure of her future emotions and guarantee that her attitude to her child by an unknown father forever afterwards will be appropriate. It will not be the child of her husband. It could hardly have been conceived in love, as a child should be, although love may come with birth, but love could also come with adoption.

It may be said that this reasoning gives us no clear, precise, moral command. That should not be surprising. We are dealing with a subject so extremely delicate and so deeply complex. But in spite of that, I will venture to summarise. I cannot but feel that religion should sanction artificial insemination from a husband. In the remaining cases, artificial insemination by a donor only for the maintenance of esteem or for deceptive purposes or for merely personal satisfaction, must be condemned without qualification. Artificial insemination from a donor, where husband and wife agree, involves so much that is questionable and at this stage incalculable, that I think it should be in the main definitely discouraged. In many of its aspects it is not compatible with the divine sanctity of the human personality.

I know that this may be said to be a gospel of austerity but it may be that in no range of life can we escape a certain austerity. The war is really the product of international anarchy and peace will only be won under the sternest discipline. In a very real sense we can enter life only with a cross on our backs, yet by itself, this would be a false presentation of the case. It would be giving priority to the secondary, for such is the grace of God, such its amazing transforming power, that man can be the master of his nature and his circumstances, and one cannot but strongly assert that before the grave disappointments and deep tragedies of human life there is in the will of Christ a healing light and an overcoming power.

SUMMING UP BY THE CHAIRMAN

THE RIGHT HON. VISCOUNT CALDECOTE, C.B.E., K.C., LL.D.

I WANT to thank the speakers who have illuminated this problem from their own experience. I came into this room as a learner and I have been astonished to hear that this practice has been so widespread, not in this country but in America. It has gone a great deal further there than in this country. I think the Public Morality Council, under whose auspices we are meeting, is to be congratulated on arranging this discussion. I heard from Mr. Willink, who was to have spoken here, that he is serving on the Archbishop's Commission to inquire into the whole subject and to report. I think it is a subject on which, if we profess Christian ideals, we ought to be very careful indeed, about anything we say about people's opinions on this question. I was rather horrified to hear what Dr. Barton said, that people are to be found who charge the doctors with thinking in terms of personal advantage or wealth in this matter. That should never be done.

I am asked to sum up this discussion and I really do not feel that I am qualified to do so. Various aspects of this question have been mentioned and I am sure that the Public Morality Council and its advisers can formulate opinions upon it without the help of someone who is really a tyro. I think that this problem will acquire greater importance and that the questions involved will be recognised. I do not speak with any knowledge about the question of artificial insemination but I do know a little about adoption and I have been struck throughout the proceedings with the similarity of the problems involved. The husband's consent must, of course, be secured in every adoption case. That is to say, the consent of the husband or the would-be-father to have a child brought into the family life must be obtained and those familiar with the work of the adoption associations know how successful the majority of adoptions are.

One speaker referred to the necessity for secrecy. I rather feel that that is something which may be treated as a pointer. If something must be kept secret it is probably wrong, I am rather of that view to-night. I feel that the whole question is one of real difficulty. I have known many childless couples and I think the condition of these people is to be deplored and that everything should be done for them. With these rather unhelpful observations I think I may now conclude the discussion.

Printed in Dunstable, United Kingdom

91221463R00057